MEDICARE MADNESS

BY

RICHARD E. MAXWELL

MEDICARE MADNESS

TABLE OF CONTENTS

MEDICARE MADNESS

MEDICARE MADNESS

INTRODUCTION

On July 30, 1965 the amended Social Security Act was signed into law by President Lyndon B. Johnson. The first person to be a beneficiary of the act was former President Harry S. Truman and his wife Bess was the second beneficiary. At the signing the average lifespan for our citizens was 73 for females and 66 for males. According to the 2010 Census Statistical Abstract the average lifespan is now 81 for females and 76 for males, in other words since its signing we now live almost 10 years longer then when the act was created. This is only one aspect of the financial problem that we are having with the social entitlements in the United States. The other aspects are: Number of workers vs. number of beneficiaries; increased medical costs; Medicare Taxes, other persons who are allowed to use Medicare services; fraud and waste.

In this book I will attempt to show the cost impact from the increased lifespan and the other factors effecting this entitlement.

MEDICARE MADNESS

CHAPTER 1
BACKGROUND ON MEDICARE

Shortly following the assassination of President Kennedy, Vice-President Lyndon B. Johnson was sworn in as President. On November 22, 1963 after assuming the Presidential reins and settling into his power position President Johnson introduced a socialist program entitled *The Great Society.* A part of that program was called, *The War on Poverty* which included an amendment to the Social Security Act, which is now known as Medicare and Medicaid.

On July 30, 1965 when President Lyndon B. Johnson signed the Medicare Amendment to the Social Security Act there were less than 20,000,000 citizens aged over 65 and the life expectancy was less than 75 for a female and less than 69 for a male. The law was financed by payroll taxes of 2.9% split evenly between the worker and the employer. There was a maximum amount of payroll that would be taxed under the law.

You may believe that the requirement to be eligible to be a beneficiary of Medicare was your age. You are wrong if this is your belief. The rules are:

The Medicare Part A premiums are entirely waived if you are 65 years or older and have been a permanent legal resident for 5 continuous years and they or their spouse has paid Medicare taxes for at

MEDICARE MADNESS

least 10 years, or;

You are under 65, disabled and have been receiving either Social Security SSDI benefits or Railroad Retirement Board disability benefits. They must have been receiving one of these benefits for at least 24 months from the date of receiving the first disability payment before becoming eligible to enroll in Medicare, or;

They get continuing dialysis for end stage renal disease or need a kidney transplant, or;

They are eligible for Social Security Disability Insurance and have amyotrophic lateral sclerosis (ALS or known as Lou Gehrig's disease), or

Many beneficiaries are dual-eligible and can qualify for Medicare and Medicaid. In some states for those making below a certain income, Medicaid will pay the beneficiaries Part B premium for them.

In 1966, the first year of enrollment for Medicare, there were 19,100,000 elderly (over 65 years of age) enrolled in Medicare with no non-elderly disabled (under age 65) in the plan. In 2008 Medicare provided healthcare coverage for 45,000,000, including 7,500,000 non-elderly Americans at a cost in access of $450,000,000,000 from a trust fund containing around $460,000,000,000. Does this show you anything?

MEDICARE MADNESS

The cost of Medicare doubled every four years between 1966 and 1980 and that was before the Baby Boomers started reaching retirement age. Look at the following chart.

Baby Boomer Chart*

Age Bracket	Born	Number
54 - 57	1946 - 1949	13,543,850
49 - 53	1950 - 1954	19,331,673
44 - 48	1955 - 1959	21,891,470
39 - 43	1960 - 1964	23,005,812
Total		77,705,865

During this period the birthrate was above 2.1 to the total population. Shortly following the 1960 decade the birthrate dropped below 2.0 and in 2000 it was 1.4.

For those of you not knowing who the Baby Boomers are I will furnish you an explanation: During World War II, which was mainly fought by males aged 18 to 35, many of whom were drafted into the military service. These males were away from their families for extended periods of time and therefore were not in the United States during their most reproductive period. Upon their return there was a large increase in marriage and a large increase of child birth following the end of the war. This continued during the period of the Korean and Viet Nam wars which also had the draft still existing. Those born in 1946 reach the age of 65 in 2011. To show the impact of the "Boomers" to you here is some data: In 1940 the number of babies born in the United States was 2,360,000; ten years later the number of babies born was 3,632,000 or an increase of 54% over 1940. This was merely an indication since in 1960 there were 4,258,000 babies born or an increase of 80% over 1940. Do you now understand why they were called "Baby Boomers"?

As a summary of this first chapter, that explains the beginning of Medicare, here is the data:

> Medicare began in 1965 with $999,000,000 paid by the government to insure 19,100,000 beneficiaries the first year of coverage in the plan in 1966.

> The initial amount of money paid into the Medicare Trust Fund was $1,943,000,000This leaves a surplus in the fund of $944,000,000.

> All of the beneficiaries the first year were seniors over 65 years of age.

> In 1966 there was an estimated 5 employed persons per beneficiary.

In future chapters I will provide you the data to show you how these Baby Boomer beneficiaries effect the cost of Medicare.

MEDICARE MADNESS

CHAPTER 2
OUTLIVING COVERAGE

When Medicare began in 1965 there were less than 20,000,000 citizens aged over 65 and the life expectancy was less than 75 for a female and less than 69 for a male. The next data section will show the change in the average life span for our residents and after the data table I will bring to your attention some of the reasons for the dramatic change. Please review this chart:

LIFE EXPECTANCY*

Decade	Female	Male
1920	58	54
1940	65	61
1960	73	66
1980	76	70
2000	79.5	74.1
2010	80.8	75.7

* Statistical *abstract of US Census*

By reviewing the 1920 decade you see that the average lifespan of both females and males was in the mid 50's and by the 1960 decade the lifespan had risen by over 12 years. You would have thought that the planners of Medicare would have been aware of this increase and would have thought that this would continue. An increase has continued but at a rate of 50 percent of the 1920 to 1960 period. The next period in the Life Expectancy chart, from the 2000 decade to the 2010 decade has continued the reduced

MEDICARE MADNESS

rate. This shows you that longer lifespan is a factor in the financial burden, even though it is not growing as rapidly as previous. Next I will show you another factor that enters the equation, and that is the average medical expense paid each year per beneficiary.

In the initial implementation year of Medicare, 1966, the average annual expense for each of the 19,100,000 beneficiaries was $5,230. This is a total of $999,000 Medicare expense. In 2009, the last year for which data is available there were 46,100,000 beneficiaries and the average expense per year was $10,842 making a total Medicare expense of $499,837,000,000.

In viewing the data in these last two paragraphs you will see that the average lifespan has increased by at least 11%, the number of beneficiaries has more than doubled, and the average annual expenditure per beneficiary has also more than doubled. Now let us look at a hypothetical lady who became a beneficiary in 2010 and lived to the age of 81. If she received the average 2009 annual Medicare of $10,842 and the total expenditure will end up being $173,472.

Another aspect of the dramatic increase in spending for Medicare is the sizable increase in beneficiaries of the coverage. In a previous paragraph I showed that in 1966 there were 19,100,000 beneficiaries

MEDICARE MADNESS

signed up for the benefits. In the year 2010 there were 47,000,000 persons signed up to receive benefits, that is an increase of 2.46 times the original number, and that does not include the Baby Boomers who begin retirement in 2011. Please review the following chart:

NATIONAL INSTITUTE ON AGING
OVER 65 ESTIMATES*

YEAR	OVER 65 POPULATION
2000**	35,000,000**
2005**	37,000,000**
2010	40,229,000
2015	45,200,000
2020	53,000,000
2025	61,000,000
2030	66,000,000
2035	70,500,000
2040	76,000,000
2045	80,000,000
2050	83,500,000

*8/6/09 from Census population projection
** actual

This chart shows the anticipated increase in the over 65 population projected to the year 2050. This chart only shows beneficiaries that are over 65 years of age. That is not all of the beneficiaries receiving Medicare. Since 1975 there are persons classified as Non-elderly Disabled and they are under age 65. In 1975 there were 2,200,000 of these under age 65

MEDICARE MADNESS

persons receiving Medicare benefits. In 2010 there were 8,000,000 such persons receiving the benefits. That is 17% of all beneficiaries, and an increase of 2.6 times as many since 1980. They have to be added to this chart, thereby increasing the recipient percentage by 17%. We are at a point now where unless modifications are made **NOW** Medicare will go bankrupt. Here is what will happen in 2015: In that year there will be 48,364,000 Medicare beneficiaries, and if we use the same average expense per beneficiary based upon the year 2009 rate of $10,842 the expense, adjusted using the same growth rate as in the 21st century, will be $683,528,000,000. If the Medicare income continues to increase at the same rate as it has in the 21st century it will be $680,960,000,000 in 2015. Where will the additional $2,568,000,000 come from?

I have shown you several sets of government charts that allow me to use their data to make my case. Now I will furnish you some of my personal data to support my views: From 2000 through 2010 my wife and I have had $165,654.58 in approved Medicare expenses covering prescriptions, doctor bills and hospital bills. That comes to an average of $16,565 per year and we are both relatively healthy with no major problems like Diabetes, etc. This is an average of $8,783 for each of us and is slightly less than the $10,842 average shown in the previous paragraph.

MEDICARE MADNESS

The Non-elderly Disabled are one of the reasons for the rapid movement of Medicare towards bankruptcy. You might ask, why do these people get their medical expenses paid by Medicare, aren't they eligible for Medicaid? Here is what the US Department of CMS Medicare and Medicaid Services has to say about this: "Many groups of people are covered by **Medicaid**. Even within these groups, though, certain requirements must be met. These may include your age, whether you are pregnant, disabled, blind, or aged;

your income and resources (like bank accounts, real property, or other items that can be sold for cash); and whether you are a U.S. citizen or a lawfully admitted immigrant. The rules for counting your income and resources vary from state to state and from group to group. There are special rules for those who live in nursing homes and for disabled children living at home."

Keep in mind that the average yearly payout has more than doubled since the law was signed into existence. When this is added to the increased lifespan it puts a heavy strain on the trust fund driving it toward bankruptcy. In the paragraph on page 8 you will see the estimated Medicare income of $680,960,000,000. That is based upon a

MEDICARE MADNESS

continuation of Medicare taxes paid by a growing number of workers. The next chapter will show you that this is unlikely to happen.

MEDICARE MADNESS

CHAPTER 3
LAW OF DIMINISHING RETURNS

As you can see, from the previous chapters Medicare is in deep financial trouble. The Baby Boomers begin to retire this year and they will increase the number of Medicare beneficiaries by 18% in the years 2011 - 2014, 68% in the years 2015 - 2018. These percentages will accelerate the following 8 years. To add to the Baby Boomer problem, our number of workers, paying Medicare taxes is declining also. Please review the following table:

Number of Workers per Medicare Beneficiary *

Year	Workers
1966	5.0
1980	7.4
1990	3.4
2000	3.4
2010	3.4
2020	2.8**
2030	2.3**

* Statistical *abstract of US Census*
** *estimate*

You will notice that in 1966, the first year anyone became eligible for Medicare, that there were 5 workers for each Medicare beneficiary. This was a period approaching the end of the Viet Nam War so this was a time of relatively high employment. If you notice the 1980 period the number of workers per beneficiary increased almost 50%. If this high

MEDICARE MADNESS

ratio of workers per beneficiary had continued we would probably not be having the funding problem that we are now. Hold on, it is going to become worse. Look at the following table:

OVER 65 POPULATION RATIO*			
DECADE	POPULATION	OVER 65	RATIO
1965	194,303,000	19,100,000	09.8%
1980	227,726,000	28,540,000	11.3%
1990	249,973,000	34,284,000	12.5%
2000	281,425,000	34,992,000	12.4%
2010	310,333,000	40,229,000	13.0%

* Statistical *abstract of US Census*

In 1965, the year that Medicare was signed into law by President Johnson, there were only 19,100,000 persons who were over 65 and eligible for Medicare. That was less than 10% of our population at that time. If we look at 1980 you will see that there was almost a 50 percent increase of the over 65's. That was still manageable, but it should have been a strong signal, had our elected officials paid any attention. In 2010 the portion of our population over age 65 has continued to grow to where it has more than doubled in the forty five years since Medicare was signed into law. In 2010 it was 13% of our population, and the Baby Boomers will begin to be over 65 in one more year. 2011.

The data shown in this chapter shows the stress that is being put on Medicare by the increasing number of beneficiaries receiving coverage and the reduced

MEDICARE MADNESS

percentage of workers paying into the Medicare fund. When this is added to the fact that the average lifespan is at least 11% longer than it was in 1965, which is 11 years, and growing. In 2009 the average yearly payout per beneficiary was $12,495 when multiplied by the 11 years of average increase in lifespan equals to an increased payout of $137,495 per beneficiary. When the arithmetic is done this means there will be an average increase in total Medicare expenses per year of $502,000. How long do you feel we can afford this without going broke. In 2010 the income and payout for Medicare was almost equal. Again, this does not take into consideration the Baby Boomers.

In order to see the impact caused by these increases this next chart will furnish you a base from which to begin. You can use the data furnished in the first part of this chapter to see the extent of the disaster that we are headed toward.

MEDICARE ENROLEES*

DECADE	ENROLEES	CHANGE
1980	28,500,000	
1990	34,200,000	+0.2 %
2000	39,700,000	+0.16%
2009	46,100,000	+0.16%

* Statistical *abstract of US Census*

MEDICARE MADNESS

In addition to the reduction of workers per Medicare beneficiary if you compare the number of over 65 beneficiaries with the number of Medicare Enrollees you will see that there are 5,183,000 people receiving benefits who have a disability which makes them eligible under the law as it is currently written. The average Medicare expense, just for these disabled beneficiaries amounts to at least $64,762,115,000.

Now let us add in the effect that the Baby Boomers will have on the Medicare expenses, beginning this year, 2011. In 2008 there were 45,412,000 persons receiving benefits, from 2000 to 2008 the average increase in persons receiving benefits was 81,741 per year. With the same increase occurring for the next two years that makes the number of beneficiaries increase to 45,575,000. Now if you review the beginning of this chapter, you will see that the effect of the Baby Boomers from 2011 to 2014 is an increase of 18% for that period. Doing the mathematics shows an estimated increase from 45,575,000 to 47,626,000 in 2011. I wish to remind you that this is the smallest effect by the Baby Boomers since in the period from 2015 to 2018 the total increase is 68%.

Do I have your attention?

CHAPTER 4
EFFECT OF VOLUNTARY BIRTH CONTROL

If you review the next data that I am including in this chapter you will see that in 1945 there were 2,858,000 child births in the United States for the entire year and our total population in 1945 was 132,481,000. If you look at the number of child births in 2010 you will see that there were 2,237,290 children born to 308,746,000 residents of the United States. That is over 620,000 fewer child births than there were 65 years earlier. You might ask what does this have to do with Medicare? Each of these children should become workers and pay a percentage of their income into the Medicare fund. The fund from which the Medicare benefits are paid is supposed to be kept solvent by Medicare Taxes paid into the fund by workers.

In 2008 you have seen that there were 45,412,000 persons receiving Medicare Benefits. Let us assume that there will not be an increase in Medicare Beneficiaries from the 2008 level and likewise assume that the number of babies born in 2010 will all grow up and become dedicated workers. Shall we do the arithmetic again, each of the 2,237,290 persons, born in 2010 and thereafter will have to pay half of the Medicare Benefits for a person receiving those benefits. Does this make any sense to you?
Do you now see why Medicare is rapidly becoming Bankrupt?

MEDICARE MADNESS

ANNUAL AND AVERAGE BIRTH RATE

YEAR OR YEARS	BIRTHS OR AVERAGE BIRTHS	%
1945	2,858,000	---
1946 - 1949	3,386,000 (avg)	+.18
1950 - 1954	4,833,000 (avg)	+.69
1955 - 1959	5,473,000 (avg)	+.91
1960 - 1964	5,751,000 (avg)	+1.01
1965 - 1969	3,601,000 (avg)	+ .63
1970 - 1974	3,392,000 (avg)	+ .94
1975 - 1979	3,360,000 (avg)	+ . 99
1980 - 1984	3,628,000 (avg)	+1.08
1985 - 1989	3,820,000 (avg)	+1.05
1990 - 1994	4,072,000 (avg)	+1.07
1995 - 1999	3,903,000 (avg)	+.958
2000 - 2004	4,074,000 (avg)	+1.04
2005 - 2009	4,242,000 (avg)	+1.04
2010	2,237,290	+ .52

When you compare my data, which came from the federal government statistics, you can see that each chapter makes the previous data worse. For instance look back at chapter 3 and you will see that in 2009 each beneficiary is having $12,495 paid on their behalf for Medicare Benefits. When I was working I was employed for 42 years and that is more time than many people work. If each worker must pay half of the benefits for each beneficiary, and it does not increase. They will have to pay $262,185 throughout their career.

We know that the cost of benefits will increase, don't we?

MEDICARE MADNESS

We have caused this to happen by ourselves. Keep in mind that this chapter is devoted to the reduction in the number of children born versus the longer lifespan that we are living. In my book, "United States - Self Destruction", I mention some of the reasons for this, and they are the result of:

☐ A dramatic drop in live births, that began in the 1980's;
☐ A large number of abortions, that also began to increase in the 1980's;

These two negatives are somewhat balanced by two positives, that are also mentioned in my book:

☐ As of 2003 the life expectancy has increased from 65 for females and 61 for males in 1960's to 80 for females and 75 for males in 2003;
☐ Our population would have not increased if it were not for immigration, mainly Hispanic which has increased by over 19,000,000 from 2000 through 2004. This does not include all of those here illegally.

When you compare these two competing situations, think about their impact on our country.

Since we are not raising enough children, who will become tax paying workers, to pay for the politically established benefits for our old age, some of this will be offset by the increase of immigration, if they pay taxes.

MEDICARE MADNESS

Unfortunately most, if not all, of this will be offset by the longer lifespan.

Have I made an explanation about this portion of the problem? Keep in mind that this does not take into consideration the impact of the "Baby Boomers".

MEDICARE MADNESS

CHAPTER 5
INCOME VERSUS OUTGO

When you are planning to purchase something, if you are a responsible money manager, you plan for the expense ahead of time, unless you are super wealthy. You likewise may have expenses that are unanticipated, for which a responsible money manager will establish a savings account in preparation for such expense. Even with such planning, you may very well have an expense that will be greater than anticipated, in which case you will have to cut back on discretionary spending. When you review the next set of tables, you will see that Medicare is rapidly moving into that category. This first chart shows Medicare expenses from it's origin through 2009.

MEDICARE EXPENSES*

DECADE	EXPENSES	CHANGE
1966	$ 999,000,000	---
1980	$ 37,500,000,000	+37.54%
1990	$109,709,000,000	+ 2.93%
2000	$219,276,000,000	+ 2.00%
2009	$499,837,000,000	+ 2.23%

* Statistical *abstract of US Census*

With the number of Medicare enrollees increasing, you would expect the expenses to increase, but in looking at the data shown in this chart are you not surprised that in the first 9 years from the year 2000

MEDICARE MADNESS

the expenses have more than doubled, especially since the number of enrollees has risen by only 16%. The reason mainly is that our elected congress has expanded the number of people receiving the benefits as was explained in chapter 3. With this in mind, shall we now review the next chart?

MEDICARE TRUST FUNDS INCOME*

DECADE	INCOME	CHANGE
1966	$ 1,943,000,000	---
1980	$ 26,097,000,000	+13.43%
1990	$126,300,000,000	+ 4.84%
2000	$257,100,000,000	+ 2.04%
2009	$511,400,000,000	+ 1.99%

* Statistical *abstract of US Census*

While there is still more income than outgo, the surplus has continued to decrease. The income is increasing by less than 2% while the expenses are increasing by more than 2%. If modifications to either the income or outgo are not made soon, the Medicare plan will be bankrupt, and then it will require massive changes. Let us now review the income and expense per Medicare enrollee.

MEDICARE MADNESS

INCOME PER ENROLEE*

DECADE	TOTAL INCOME	TOTAL ENROLLEES	INCOME PER ENROLLEE
1980	$ 26,097,000,000	28,500,000	$ 915.68
1990	$126.300,000,000	34,200,000	$ 4,210.00
2000	$257,100,000,000	39,700,000	$ 6,476.07
2009	$511,400,000,000	45,400,000	$11,262.32

* Statistical *abstract of US Census*

MEDICARE EXPENSE PER ENROLEE*

DECADE	TOTAL EXPENSE	TOTAL ENROLLEES	EXPENSE PER ENROLLEE
1980	$ 25,577,000,000	28,500,000	$ 897.44
1990	$109,709,000,000	34,200,000	$ 3,210.00
2000	$219,276,000,000	39,700,000	$ 6,000.00
2009	$499,837,000,000	45,400,000	$ 11,010.00

* Statistical *abstract of US Census*

As you can see by reviewing these two charts the average income and expense is extremely close, so there is not enough excess money to provide for changes in either beneficiaries or coverage. In the next chapter I will furnish you an estimated summery of the effects of the first five chapters.

MEDICARE MADNESS

CHAPTER 6
HERE ARE THE TOTALS

In Chapter 1, in addition to the history of Medicare I gave you a summary of the beginning of the Baby Boom Generation. It is just starting in 2011 with the first wave of Boomers beginning to retire. During the next 4 years the leading edge (over 2,600,000) will begin to retire, followed in the next 18 years by 28,000,000 additional Boomers. To make sure that you are not being misled, the average increase in childbirth from 1946 to 1964 was 31,000,000. This is calculated by subtracting the average number of child births during the years prior to 1946 from the total number of Baby Boomers, as reported by the federal government. The 31,000,000 multiplied by the average Medicare expense per beneficiary in 2009 of $11,010 equals $3,413,100,000. This when added to the 2009 Medicare total expense greatly reduces the surplus.

In Chapter 2, I showed you that the average person is now living at least 11% longer than they did when Medicare was started. That is an average of approximately 8 years of additional Medicare expense that we have as of now, and it is continuing to increase each year. If we do the arithmetic this comes out as $499,837,000,000 x 8 equals $3,998,696,000,000.

MEDICARE MADNESS

In Chapter 3, I showed you that the number of workers per Medicare Beneficiary has declined dramatically, in fact it is reducing by an average of 17% in the period from 2010. This means there are fewer persons paying Medicare taxes. In 2009 there were 45,400,000 persons paying Medicare taxes in 2009. The taxes paid were $11,262.32 per year. Assuming that there were still the same number enrolled in 2010, the 17% reduction amounts to 7,718,000 fewer persons paying Medicare taxes in 2011 than there were in 2010. This amounts to $86,729,116,000 in reduced Medicare taxes.

In Chapter 4, I showed you the effect of the declining birthrate, which has a delayed effect on the number of workers. In fact from the 1965 - 1969 period, when the Medicare Act was put into effect, we have produced 48% fewer live births in 2010. We are not producing enough baby's to keep our population growing. The only reason that it is growing is because of immigration, Legal and Illegal.

In Chapter 5, I showed you that the funds entering Medicare are rapidly declining with an average of $32,000,000 more funds being spent than are being put into the fund. If this rate continues it will exhaust the fund by around 2014 by itself. This will happen without the effects that I am going to cover now.

MEDICARE MADNESS

Now we will begin the summary, first the Baby Boomer Effect:

During the era from 1946 to 1964 the increase in child birth was approximately 54% more than in previous years. That means that just in 2011 alone we can expect to have an increase of at least 1,070,000 retirees bringing the total number of Medicare Beneficiaries to over 46,000,000. If we continue to spend at the same rate as 2009, $11,010.00 per enrollee, then the addition of 1,070,000 more members increases the Medicare expenses by $11,781,000,000 or a total of $514,813,000,000. (that is just during the years from 2011 through 2015. Keep in mind this is an annual expense. This $514,813,000,000 will have to be spent for at least 8 additional years, as caused by the increased life span that was discussed in chapter 2.

Next we must consider that during the next 9 years there will continue to be a gradual 17% reduction of workers paying into the Medicare system. The tax rate paid, including employee and employer, is 2.9% on total salary. If a working person is being paid the salary that is the same as the average paid in 2009, the Medicare tax paid by both the employee and the employer would be $1.061.23 per employee, if being paid at the average. During the next 9 years we will see the 17% reduction in workers take place and that will generate reduction of $134,800,000,000

MEDICARE MADNESS

in Medicare revenue to be coupled with the increase of $11,010.00 per enrollee. This was discussed in Chapter 3. We cannot be real accurate in this projection since what is occurring now is affected by immigration, if they are legally working, plus the fact that we are projecting based on past performance.. The reduced birthrate, as shown in chapter 4 is the main cause for this problem.

Keep in mind the gradual decline in funds entering the Medicare system, as was discussed in chapter 5. Do you now see why I am concerned with the future of Medicare?

MEDICARE MADNESS

CHAPTER 7
WHEN WILL MEDICARE GO BROKE?

In chapter 6 I gave you my best estimates, of the deficits, as we are currently (as of 2011) proceeding. In this final chapter I will do my best to sum them all up for you.

DEFICITS

Baby Boomer effect, by 2029	- $ 3,413,100,000
Longer lifespan as of now	- $ 3,498,859,000
Reduced number of workers	- $ 86,729,116,000
(Fewer babies being born	
Included in reduced workers)	
Yearly Spending more	
than receiving	- $ 32,000,000
Total	- $ 93,673,075,000

This total is 18.3% of the total receipts by Medicare in 2009. You do not have to be an accountant to see that we are rapidly going broke. In fact it may occur before 2014 as I had estimated in chapter 6.

Now please notice that this is regarding Medicare not Medicaid!

One of the Republican candidates for president stated that Social Security and Medicare is a Ponzi Scheme. He should have explained what he meant. The reason that they can be considered as a Ponzi Scheme, is not because of the plans

MEDICARE MADNESS

themselves, it is because of the way that they are setup and the fact that the money that is supposed to be in a "lock box" has been spent by the congress, who replaced the funds with promissory notes. With the current state of our spending I do not believe the money will be there when the notes come due. That is a Ponzi Scheme, not the plans.

By the way, I am 80 years of age as I am writing this, so my wife and I will be affected by this Ponzi Scheme.